THE COOKBOOK FOR YOUR LEAN AND GREEN DIET

50 delicious and easy to prepare recipes for your lean and green diet, to stay fit and boost energy

Josephine Reed

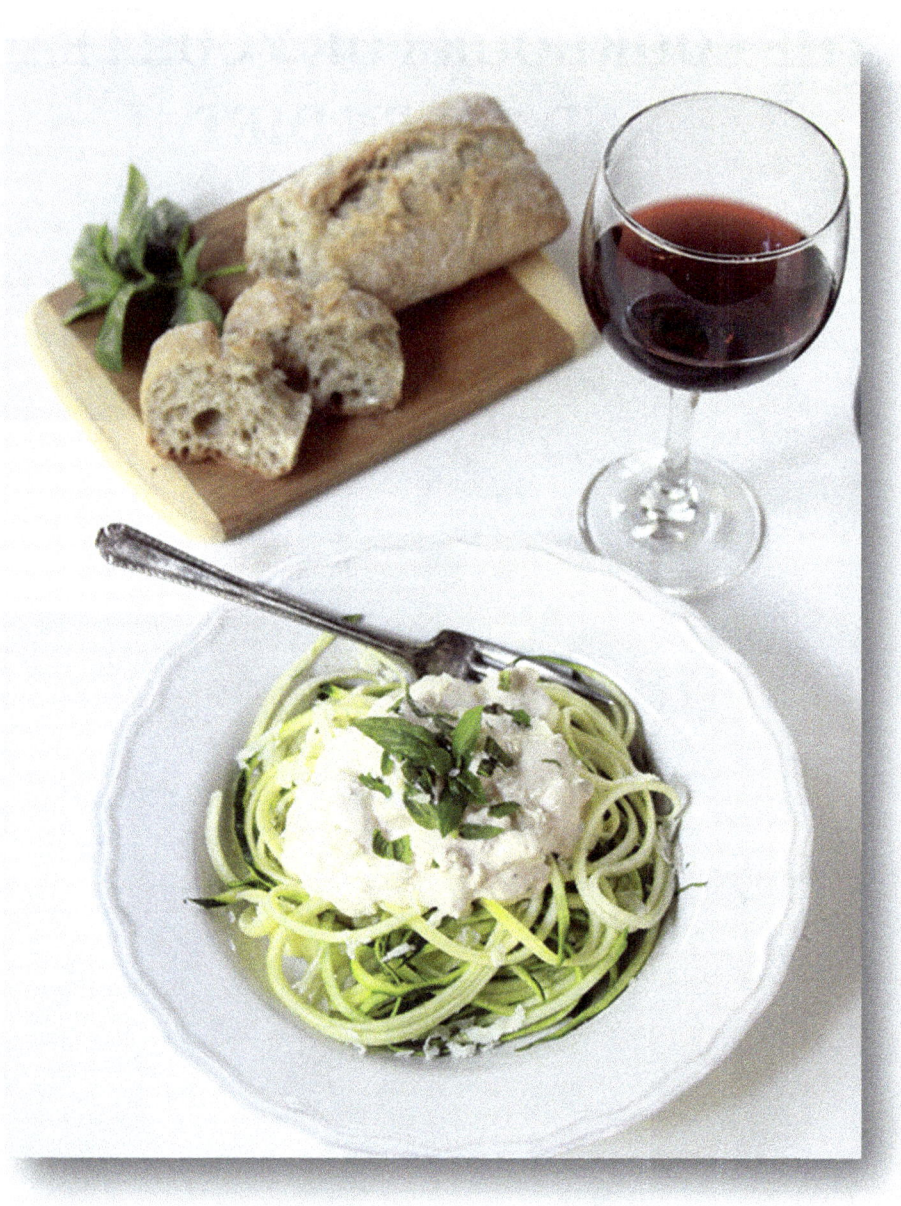

© Copyright 2021 - All rights reserved.

The content contained within this book may not be reproduced, duplicated or transmitted without direct written permission from the author or the publisher.

Under no circumstances will any blame or legal responsibility be held against the publisher, or author, for any damages, reparation, or monetary loss due to the information contained within this book. Either directly or indirectly.

Legal Notice:

This book is copyright protected. This book is only for personal use. You cannot amend, distribute, sell, use, quote or paraphrase any part, or the content within this book, without the consent of the author or publisher.

Disclaimer Notice:

Please note the information contained within this document is for educational and entertainment purposes only. All effort has been executed to present accurate, up to date, and reliable, complete information. No warranties of any kind are declared or implied. Readers acknowledge that the author is not engaging in the rendering of legal, financial, medical or professional advice. The content within this book has been derived from various sources.

Please consult a licensed professional before attempting any techniques outlined in this book.

By reading this document, the reader agrees that under no circumstances is the author responsible for any losses, direct or indirect, which are incurred as a result of the use of information contained within this document, including, but not limited to, — errors, omissions, or inaccuracies.

Table of contents

Chicken, Cucumber & Tomato Salad 8
Chicken, Kale & Olives Salad 10
Chicken, Kale & Cucumber Salad 12
Turkey & Veggie Salad 15
Ground Turkey Salad 17
Steak & Tomato Salad 20
Steak, Egg & Veggies Salad 22
Steak & Kale Salad 24
Steak & Veggie Salad 26
Chicken & Bell Pepper Muffins 28
Chicken & Kale Muffins 30
Eggs with Kale & Tomatoes 32
Eggs with Veggies 35
Chicken & Veggie Frittata 37
Broccoli Frittata 39
Chicken & Veggie Quiche 41
Kale & Mushroom Frittata 43
Kale & Bell Pepper Frittata 45
Mushroom & Tomato Omelet 47
Tomato & Egg Scramble 50
Tofu & Spinach Scramble 52
Tofu & Veggie Scramble 54
Chicken & Zucchini Pancakes 55

Broccoli Waffles	57
Cheesy Spinach Waffles	58
Pesto Zucchini Noodles	60
Baked Cod & Vegetables	62
Parmesan Zucchini	64
Chicken Zucchini Noodles	66
Tomato Cucumber Avocado Salad	68
Creamy Cauliflower Soup	70
Taco Zucchini Boats	72
Healthy Broccoli Salad	74
Delicious Zucchini Quiche	76
Turkey Spinach Egg Muffins	78
Chicken Casserole	80
Shrimp Cucumber Salad	82
Asparagus & Shrimp Stir Fry	84
Turkey Burgers	86
Broccoli Kale Salmon Burgers	88
Pan Seared Cod	90
Quick Lemon Pepper Salmon	91
Healthy Salmon Salad	93
Pan Seared Tilapia	96
Creamy Broccoli Soup	97
Tuna Muffins	99
Chicken Cauliflower Rice	101
Easy Spinach Muffins	103
Healthy Cauliflower Grits	105

Spinach Tomato Frittata..107

Chicken, Cucumber & Tomato Salad

Prep Time: 15 minutes

Cook Time: 16 minutes

Serve: 4

Ingredients:

- 4 (6-ounce) boneless, skinless chicken breast halves
- Salt and freshly ground black-pepper, to taste 2 normale spoons olive oil
- 1 tomato, chopped
- 1 cucumber, chopped
- 3 cup fresh baby greens
- 3 cup lettuce, torn

Instructions:

1.Season each half of each chicken breast evenly with salt and black pepper.

2.Place chicken over a rack set in a rimmed baking sheet.

3.Refrigerate for at least 30 minutes.

4.Remove from refrigerator and with paper towels, pat dry the chicken breasts.

5. In a 11-inch skillet, heat the oil over medium-low heat.

6. Place the chicken breast halves, smooth-side down, and cook for about 9-10 minutes, without moving.

7. Flip the chicken breasts and cook for about 6 minutes or until cooked through.

8. Remove the skillet from heat and let the chicken stand in the pan for about 3 minutes.

9. Divide greens, lettuce, cucumber and tomatoes onto serving plates.

10. Top each plate with 1 breast half and serve.

Chicken, Kale & Olives Salad

Prep Time: 15 minutes

Serve: 4

Ingredients:

For Dressing:

- 2 tablespoons fresh orange juice
- 2 tablespoons fresh lemon juice
- 3 tablespoons extra-virgin olive oil
- 1 tablespoon red wine vinegar
- 1 tablespoon honey
- 1 tablespoon fresh orange zest, grated
- ¾ tablespoon Dijon mustard
- Salt and ground black pepper, as required

For Salad:

- 3 cups cooked chicken, chopped
- 2 cups mixed olives, pitted
- 1 cup red onion, chopped
- 6 cups fresh kale, tough ribs removed and torn

Instructions:

1. For Dressing: in a small bowl, add all ingredients and beat well.

2. For Salad: in a big-salad bowl, mix together all ingredients.

3. Place dressing over salad and toss to coat well.

Chicken, Kale & Cucumber Salad

Prep Time: 15 minutes

Cook Time: 18 minutes

Serve: 4

Ingredients:

For Chicken:

- 1 teaspoon dried thyme
- ½ teaspoon garlic powder
- ½ teaspoon onion powder
- ¼ teaspoon cayenne pepper
- ¼ teaspoon ground turmeric
- Salt and ground black pepper, as required
- 2 (7-ounce) boneless, skinless chicken breasts, pounded into ¾-inch thickness
- 1 tablespoon extra-virgin olive oil

For Salad:

- 5 cups fresh kale, tough ribs removed and chopped
- 1 cup cucumber, chopped
- ½ cup red onion, sliced
- ¼ cup pine nuts

For Dressing:

- 1 small garlic clove, minced
- 2 tablespoons fresh lemon juice
- 2 tablespoons extra-virgin olive oil
- 1 teaspoon maple syrup
- Salt and ground black pepper, as required

Instructions:

1. Preheat your oven to 429 degrees F. Line a baking dish with parchment paper.

2. For chicken: in a bowl, mix together the thyme, spices, salt and black pepper.

3. Drizzle the chicken breasts with oil and then rub with spice mixture generously and drizzle with the oil.

4. On the prepared baking platter, arrange the chicken breasts.

5. Bake for approximately 16-18 minutes.

6. Remove pan from oven and place the chicken breasts onto a cutting board for about 5 minutes.

7. For Salad: place all ingredients in a salad bowl and mix.

8. For Dressing: place all ingredients in another bowl and beat until well combined.

9. Cut each chicken breast into desired sized slices.

10. Place the salad onto each serving plate and top each with chicken slices.

11. Drizzle with dressing and serve.

Turkey & Veggie Salad

Prep Time: 15 minutes

Serve: 4

Ingredients:

For Salad:

- 3 cups cooked turkey meat, chopped
- 2 cups, cucumber, chopped
- 1 cup cherry tomatoes, halved
- 1 cup radishes, trimmed and sliced
- 6 cups fresh baby arugula
- 4 tablespoons scallion greens, chopped
- 4 tablespoons fresh parsley leaves, chopped

For Dressing:

- 1 garlic clove, minced
- 3 tablespoons extra-virgin olive oil
- 1 tablespoon balsamic vinegar
- 1 tablespoon fresh lemon juice
- Salt and ground black pepper, as required

Instructions:

1.For Salad: in a large serving bowl, add all the ingredients and mix.

2.For Dressing: in another bowl, add all the ingredients and beat till well combined.

3.Pour dressing over salad and gently toss to coat well.

Ground Turkey Salad

Prep Time: 20minutes

Cook Time: 13 minutes

Serve: 6

Ingredients:

- 1-pound ground turkey
- 1 tablespoon olive oil
- Salt and ground black pepper, as required
- ¼ cup water
- ½ of English cucumber, chopped
- 4 cups green cabbage, shredded
- ½ cup fresh mint leaves, chopped
- 2 tablespoons fresh lime juice
- ¼ cup walnuts, chopped

Instructions:

1. Heat the oil in a big-skillet over medium-high heat and cook the turkey for around 6-8 minutes, using a spatula to break up the bits.

2. Stir in the water and cook for about 4-5 minutes or until almost all the liquid is evaporated.

3.Remove from the heat and transfer the turkey into a bowl.

4.Set the bowl aside to cool completely.

5.In a big-serving bowl, add the vegetables, mint and lime juice and mix well.

6.Add the cooked turkey and stir to combine.

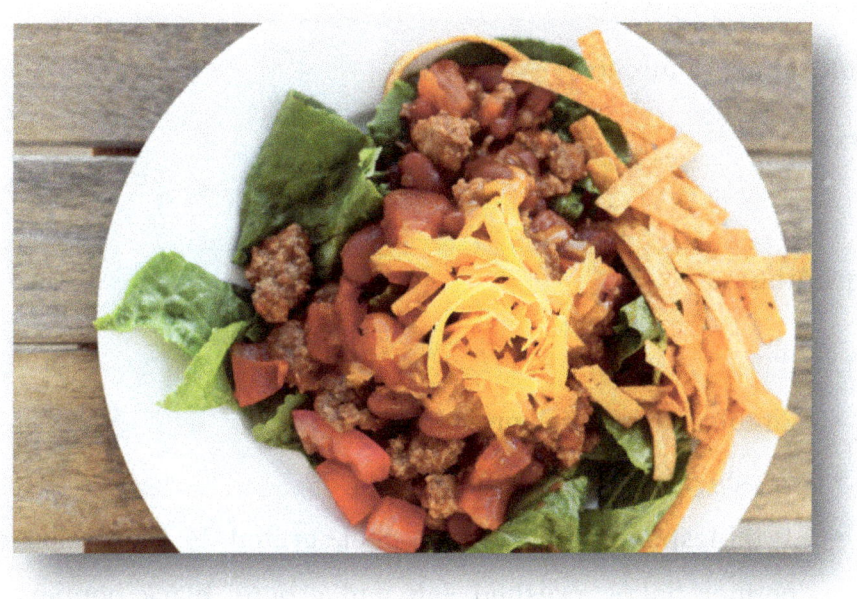

Steak & Tomato Salad

Prep Time: 15 minutes

Cook Time: 15 minutes

Serve: 5

Ingredients:

For Steak:

- 2 tablespoons fresh oregano, chopped
- ½ tablespoon garlic, minced
- 1 tablespoon fresh lemon peel, grated ½ teaspoon red pepper flakes, crushed Salt and ground black pepper, as required
- 1 (1-pound) (1-inch thick) boneless beef top sirloin steak

For Salad:

- 6 cups fresh salad greens
- 2 cups cherry tomatoes, halved
- 2 tablespoons olive oil
- 2 tablespoons fresh lime juice
- Salt and ground black pepper, as required

Instructions:

1. Preheat the gas grill to medium heat.

2. Lightly grease the grill grate.

3. For steak: in a bowl, add the oregano, garlic, lemon peel, red pepper flakes, salt and black pepper and mix well.

4. Rub the steak with garlic mixture evenly.

5. Put the steak on the grill and cook, covered, sometimes flipping, for about 12-17 minutes.

6. Remove the steak from the grill and position it for approximately 10 minutes on a cutting board.

7. Meanwhile, For Salad: in a large serving bowl, place all ingredients and toss to coat well.

8. Cut the steak into bite-sized pieces.

9. Add the steak pieces into the bowl of salad and toss to coat well.

Steak, Egg & Veggies Salad

Prep Time: 20 minutes

Cook Time: 9 minutes

Serve: 4

Ingredients:

For Steak:

- 2 tablespoons extra-virgin olive oil
- 1-pound flank steak, sliced thinly
- Salt and ground black pepper, as require

For Salad:

- 4 hard-boiled eggs, peeled and halved
- 1 cup radishes, cut into matchsticks
- 1 cup cucumber, cut into matchsticks
- 1 cup tomato, chopped
- ½ cup scallion greens, chopped

For Dressing:

- ¼ cup fresh orange juice
- 3 tablespoons extra-virgin olive oil
- 2 tablespoons low-sodium soy sauce
- 2 tablespoons white vinegar

- 1 tablespoon fresh lime juice
- 1 tablespoon maple syrup
- 1 teaspoon fresh lime zest, grated
- 1 garlic clove, minced

Instructions:

1.Heat oil in a big-heavy-bottomed pan over medium-high heat and sear the beef slices with salt and black-pepper for about 3-6 minutes or until cooked through.

2.Transfer the beef slices onto a plate and set aside.

3.Meanwhile, in a pan of the lightly salted boiling water, cook the noodles for about 5 minutes.

4.Drain well with the noodles and rinse under cold water.

5.Drain the noodles again.

6.For Dressing: in a bowl, add all ingredients and beat until well combined.

7.Divide beef slices, noodles, veggies and scallion into serving bowls and drizzle with dressing.

Steak & Kale Salad

Prep Time: 15 minutes

Cook Time: 8 minutes

Serve: 2

Ingredients:

For Steak:

- 2 teaspoons olive oil
- 2 (4-ounce) strip steaks
- Salt and ground black pepper, as required

For Salad:

- ½ cup carrot, peeled and shredded
- ½ cup cucumber, peeled, seeded and sliced
- 3 cups-fresh kale, tough ribs removed and chopped

For Dressing:

- 1 tablespoon extra-virgin olive oil
- 1 tablespoon fresh lemon juice
- Salt and ground black pepper, as required

Instructions:

1. For steak: in a large heavy-bottomed skillet, heat the oil over high heat and cook the steaks with salt and black pepper for about 3-4 minutes per side.

2. Transfer the steaks onto a cutting board for about 5 minutes before slicing.

3. For Salad: place all ingredients in a salad bowl and mix.

4. For Dressing: place all ingredients in another bowl and beat until well combined.

5. Cut the steaks into desired sized slices against the grain.

6. Place the salad onto each serving plate.

7. Top each plate with steak slices.

8. Drizzle with dressing.

Steak & Veggie Salad

Prep Time: 20 minutes

Cook Time: 16 minutes

Serve: 8

Ingredients:

For Steak:

- 2 garlic cloves, crushed
- 1 teaspoon fresh ginger, grated
- 1 tablespoon honey
- 2 normal spoons olive oil
- Salt and freshly ground black-pepper, to taste
- 1½ pounds flank steak, trimmed

For Dressing:

- 1 garlic clove, minced
- 4 tablespoons extra-virgin olive oil
- 3 tablespoons fresh lime juice
- ¼ little spoon red-pepper flakes, crushed
- Salt and freshly ground black-pepper, to taste

For Salad:

- 3 cup cucumber, sliced

- 3 cup cherry tomatoes, halved
- 1 cup red onion, sliced thinly
- 4 tablespoons fresh mint leaves
- 8 cup fresh spinach, torn

Instructions:

1.For steak: in a large sealable bag, mix together all ingredients except steak.

2.Add steak and coat with marinade generously.

3.Seal the bag and refrigerate to marinate for about 24 hours.

4.Remove from the refrigerator and set aside in room temperature for about 15 minutes.

5.Heat a Lightly-greased grill pan over-medium-high heat and cook the steak for about 6-8 minutes per side.

6.Remove the steak from grill pan and place onto a cutting board for about 10 minutes before slicing.

7.For Dressing: in a small bowl, add all ingredients and beat well.

8.For Salad: in a large-salad bowl, mix together all ingredients.

9.With a sharp knife, cut into desired slices.

10.On serving plates, divide the salad and top with steak slices.

11.Drizzle with dressing and serve immediately.

Chicken & Bell Pepper Muffins

Prep Time: 15 minutes

Cook Time: 20 minutes

Serve: 4

Ingredients:

- 8 eggs
- Salt and ground black-pepper, as required 2 tablespoons water
- 8 ounces cooked chicken, chopped finely
- 1 cup green-bell-pepper, seeded and chopped
- 1 cup onion, chopped

Instructions:

1.Preheat your oven to 350 degrees F.

2.Grease 8 cups of a muffin tin.

3.In a bowl, add eggs, black pepper and water and beat until well combined.

4.Add the chicken, bell-pepper and onion and stir to combine.

5.Transfer the mixture in prepared muffin cups evenly.

6.Bake for approximately 17-21 minutes or until golden brown.

7.Remove the muffin tin from oven and place onto a wire rack to cool for about 10 minutes.

8.Carefully invert the muffins onto a platter and serve warm.

Chicken & Kale Muffins

Prep Time: 15 minutes

Cook Time: 20 minutes

Serve: 4

Ingredients:

- 8 eggs
- Freshly ground black pepper, as required
- 2 tablespoons water
- 7 ounces cooked chicken, chopped finely
- 1½ cups fresh kale, tough ribs removed and chopped
- 1 cup onion, chopped
- 2 tablespoons fresh parsley, chopped

Instructions:

1. Preheat your oven to 350 degrees F.

2. Grease 8 cups of a muffin tin.

3. In a bowl, add eggs, black pepper and water and beat until well combined.

4. Add chicken, kale, onion and parsley and stir to combine.

5.Transfer the mixture in prepared muffin cups evenly.

6.Bake for approximately 17-21 minutes or until golden brown.

7.Remove the muffin tin from oven and place onto a wire rack to cool for about 10 minutes.

8.Carefully invert the muffins onto a platter.

Eggs with Kale & Tomatoes

Prep Time: 15 minutes

Cook Time: 25 minutes

Serve: 4

Ingredients:

- 2 tablespoons olive oil
- 1 yellow onion, chopped
- 2 garlic cloves, minced
- 1 cup tomatoes, chopped
- ½ pound fresh kale, tough ribs removed and chopped 1 teaspoon ground cumin
- ¼ teaspoon red pepper flakes, crushed
- Salt and ground black pepper, as required 4 eggs
- 2 tablespoons fresh parsley, chopped

Instructions:

1. In a large nonstick wok, heat the olive oil over medium heat and sauté the onion for about 4-5 minutes.

2. Add the garlic and sauté for approximately 1 minute.

3. Add the tomatoes, spices, salt and black pepper and cook for about 2-3 minutes, stirring frequently.

4.Attach the kale and cook for 4-5 minutes or so.

5.Carefully crack eggs on top of kale mixture.

6.With the lid, cover the wok and cook for about 10 minutes or until desired doneness of eggs.

7.Serve hot with the garnishing of parsley.

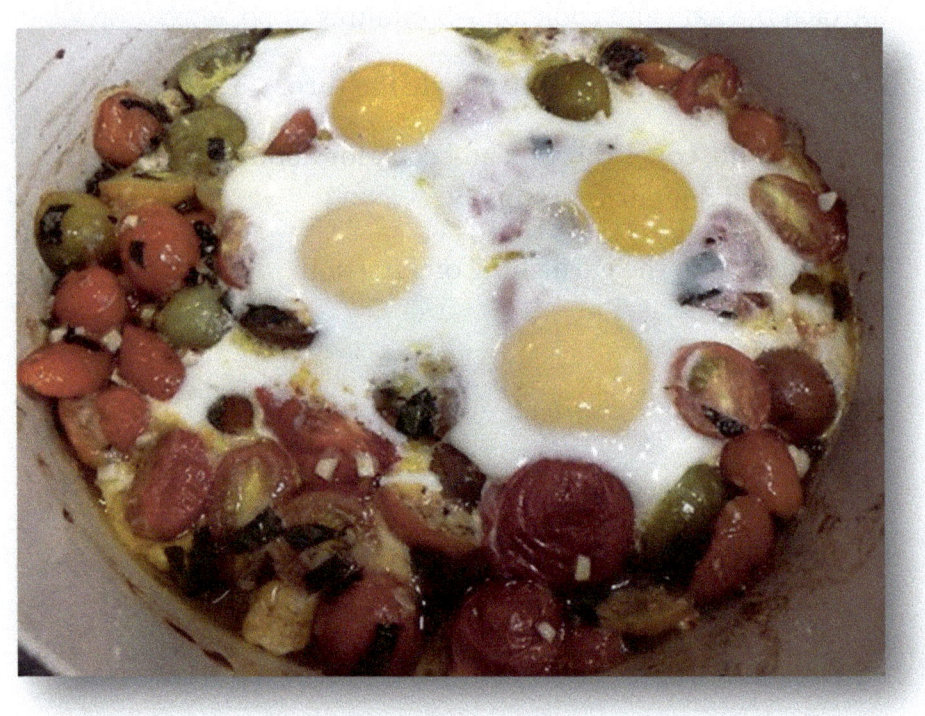

Eggs with Veggies

Prep Time: 10 minutes

Cook Time: 15 minutes

Serve: 4

Ingredients:

- 2 tablespoons olive oil, divided
- ¾ pound zucchini, quartered and sliced thinly
- 1 red bell pepper, seeded and chopped
- 1 medium onion, chopped
- 1 teaspoon fresh rosemary, chopped finely
- Salt and ground black pepper, as required 4 large eggs

Instructions:

1.In a large skillet, heat 1 tablespoon of oil over medium-high heat and sauté the zucchini, bell pepper and onion for about 5-8 minutes.

2.Add the rosemary, salt and black pepper and stir to combine.

3.With a wooden spoon, make a large well in the center of skillet by moving the veggie mixture towards the sides.

4.Reduce the heat to medium and pour the remaining oil in the well.

5.Carefully crack the eggs in the well and sprinkle the eggs with salt and black pepper.

6.Cook for about 1-2 minutes.

7.Cover the skillet and cook for about 1-2 minutes more.

8.For serving, carefully scoop the veggie mixture onto 4 serving plates.

9.Top each serving with an egg.

Chicken & Veggie Frittata

Prep Time: 45 minutes

Cook Time: 15 minutes

Serve: 8

Ingredients:

- 1 teaspoon olive oil
- ½ cup yellow onion, sliced
- 2 garlic cloves, minced
- 2 cups fresh spinach, chopped
- 1 cup red-bell-pepper, seeded and chopped
- 2 cups cooked chicken, chopped
- 2 large eggs
- 4 large egg whites
- 1¼ cups unsweetened almond milk
- 1 cup low-fat cheddar cheese, shredded Freshly ground black pepper, as required 1 tablespoon Parmesan cheese, shredded

Instructions:

1. Preheat your oven to 350 degrees F.

2. Grease a 9-inch pie plate.

3. In a skillet, heat-oil over medium heat and sauté onion and garlic for about 2-3 minutes.

4. Add spinach and bell pepper and sauté for about 1-2 minutes.

5. Stir in chicken and transfer the mixture into the prepared pie dish evenly.

6. Add eggs, egg whites, almond milk, cheddar cheese, salt, and black pepper in a mixing bowl and beat until well combined.

7. Pour egg mixture over the chicken mixture evenly and top with Parmesan cheese.

8. Bake for approximately 40 minutes or until top becomes golden brown.

9. Remove the pie-dish from oven and set aside for about 5 minutes.

10. Cut into 8 equal-sized wedges and serve.

Broccoli Frittata

Prep Time: 15 minutes

Cook Time: 13 minutes

Serve: 6

Ingredients:

- 8 eggs
- 1 tablespoon fresh cilantro, chopped
- 1 tablespoon fresh basil, chopped
- ¼ teaspoon red pepper flakes, crushed
- Salt and ground-black-pepper, as required 2 tablespoons olive oil
- 1 bunch scallions, chopped
- 1 cup broccoli, chopped finely
- ½ cup goat cheese, crumbled

Instructions:

1. Preheat the broiler of oven.

2. Arrange the upper third of the oven on a stand.

3. In a bowl, add eggs, fresh herbs, red pepper flakes, salt and black pepper and beat well.

4. In an ovenproof-skillet, heat the oil over medium heat and sauté scallion and broccoli for about 1-2 minutes.

5. Add the egg mixture over the broccoli mixture evenly and lift the edges to let the egg mixture flow underneath.

6. Cook for about 2-3 minutes.

7. Place the cheese on top in the form of dots.

8. Now, transfer the skillet under broiler and broil for about 2-3 minutes.

9. Remove the skillet from oven and set aside for about 5 minutes.

10. Cut the frittata into desired size slices and serve.

Chicken & Veggie Quiche

Prep Time: 15 minutes

Cook Time: 20 minutes

Serve: 4

Ingredients:

- 6 eggs
- ½ cup unsweetened almond milk
- Freshly ground black pepper, to taste
- 1 cup cooked chicken, chopped
- ½ cup fresh baby spinach, chopped
- ½ cup fresh baby kale, chopped
- ¼ cup fresh mushrooms, sliced
- ¼ cup green bell-pepper, seeded and chopped 1 scallion, chopped
- ¼ cup fresh cilantro, chopped
- 1 tablespoon fresh chives, minced

Instructions:

1. Preheat the oven to 400 degrees F.

2. Lightly grease a pie dish.

3.In a big-bowl, add the eggs, almond milk, salt and black pepper and beat well. Set aside.

4.In another bowl, add the chicken, vegetables, scallion and herbs and mix well.

5.Place the chicken mixture in the bottom of prepared pie dish.

6.Place the egg mixture over chicken mixture evenly.

7.Bake for approximately 20 minutes or until a toothpick inserted in the center comes out clean.

8. Take it out of the oven and set-aside for about 5-10 minutes to cool before slicing.

9.Cut into desired size wedges and serve.

Kale & Mushroom Frittata

Prep Time: 15 minutes

Cook Time: 30 minutes

Serve: 5

Ingredients:

- 8 eggs
- ½ cup unsweetened almond milk
- Salt and ground black pepper, as required
- 1 tablespoon extra-virgin olive oil
- 1 onion, chopped
- 1 garlic clove, minced
- 1 cup fresh mushrooms, chopped
- 1½ cups fresh kale, tough ribs removed and chopped

Instructions:

1. Preheat your oven to 350 degrees F.

2. In a large bowl, place the eggs, almond milk, salt and black pepper and beat well. Set aside.

3. In a large ovenproof wok, heat the oil over medium heat and sauté the onion and garlic for about 3-4 minutes.

4.Add the mushrooms, kale, salt and black pepper and cook for about 8-10 minutes.

5.Stir in the mushrooms, then cook for 3-4 minutes or so.

6.Add the kale and cook for about 5 minutes.

7.Place the egg mixture on top evenly and cook for about 4 minutes, without stirring.

8.Transfer the wok in the oven and Bake for approximately 12-15 minutes or until desired doneness.

9.Remove from the oven and place the frittata side for about 3-5 minutes before serving.

10. Cut into desired sized wedges and serve.

Kale & Bell Pepper Frittata

Prep Time: 10 minutes

Cook Time: 17 minutes

Serve: 3

Ingredients:

- 6 eggs
- Salt, as required
- 1 tablespoon olive oil
- ½ teaspoon ground turmeric
- 1 small red-bell-pepper, seeded and chopped
- 1 cup fresh kale, trimmed and chopped
- ¼ cup fresh chives, chopped

Instructions:

1.In a bowl, add the eggs and salt and beat well. Set aside.

2.In a cast-iron skillet, heat the oil over medium-low heat and sprinkle with turmeric.

3.Immediately stir in the bell pepper and kale and sauté for about 2 minutes.

4.Place the beaten eggs over bell pepper mixture evenly and immediately reduce the heat to low.

5.Cover the skillet and bake for 10-15 minutes or so.

6.Remove from the heat and set aside for about 5 minutes.

7.Cut into equal-sized wedges and serve.

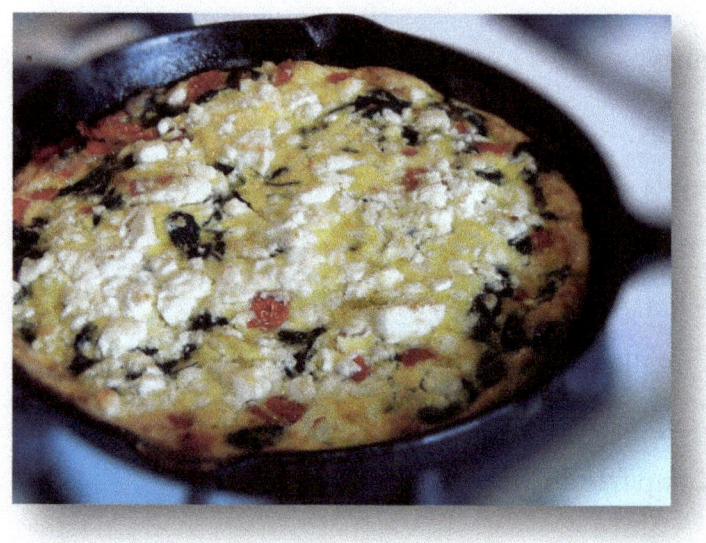

Mushroom & Tomato Omelet

Prep Time: 15 minutes

Cook Time: 36 minutes

Serve: 2

Ingredients:

- 2 poblano peppers
- Olive oil cooking spray
- 1 small tomato
- ½ teaspoon dried oregano
- ½ teaspoon chicken bouillon seasoning 4 eggs, separated
- 2 tablespoons sour cream
- ½ cup fresh white mushrooms, sliced
- 2/3 cups part-skim mozzarella cheese, shredded and divided

Instructions:

1.Preheat your oven to broiler.

2.Line a sheet with a piece of foil for baking.

3.Spray the poblano peppers with cooking spray lightly.

4. Arrange the peppers onto the prepared baking sheet in a single layer and broil for about 5-10 minutes per side or until skin becomes dark ad blistered.

5. Remove from the oven to cool and set aside.

6. After cooking, remove the stems, skin and seeds from peppers and then cut each into thin strips.

7. Meanwhile, for sauce: with a knife, make 2 small slits in a crisscross pattern on the top of tomato.

8. In a microwave-safe plate, place the tomato and microwave on High for about 2-3 minutes.

9. In a blender, add the tomato, oregano and chicken bouillon seasoning and pulse until smooth.

10. Move the sauce and set it aside in a bowl.

11. In a bowl, add the egg yolks and sour cream and beat until well combined.

12. In a clean glass bowl, add egg whites and with an electric mixer, beat until soft peaks form

13. Gently gold the egg yolk mixture into whipped egg whites

14. Heat a lightly greased skillet over medium-low heat and cook half of the egg mixture cook for about 3-5 minutes or until bottom is set

15. Place half of the mushrooms and pepper strips over one half of omelet and sprinkle with half of the cheese

16. Cover the skillet and cook for about 2-3 minutes

17. Uncover the skillet and fold in the omelet

18. Transfer the omelet onto a plate

19. Repeat with the remaining egg mixture, mushrooms, pepper strips and cheese.

20. Top each omelet with sauce.

Tomato & Egg Scramble

Prep Time: 10 minutes

Cook Time: 5 minutes

Serve: 2

Ingredients:

- 4 eggs
- ¼ teaspoon red pepper flakes, crushed Salt and ground black pepper, as required ¼ cup fresh basil, chopped
- ½ cup tomatoes, chopped
- 1 tablespoon olive oil

Instructions:

1. In a large bowl, add eggs, red pepper flakes, salt and black pepper and beat well.

2. Add the basil and tomatoes and stir to combine.

3. In a large non-stick skillet, heat th oil over medium-high heat.

4. Add the egg mixture and cook for about 3-5 minutes, stirring continuously.

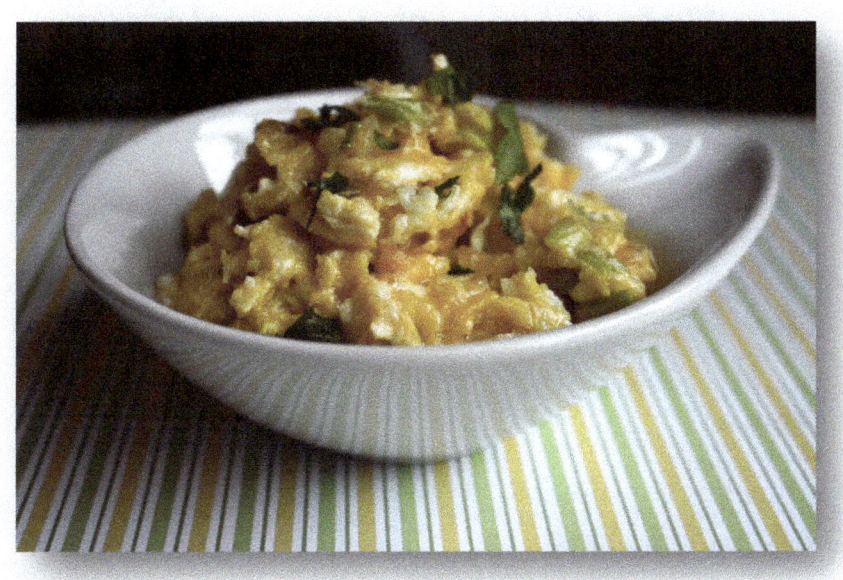

Tofu & Spinach Scramble

Prep Time: 10 minutes

Cook Time: 8 minutes

Serve: 2

Ingredients:

- 1 tablespoon olive oil
- 1 garlic clove, minced
- ¼ pound medium-firm tofu, drained, pressed and crumbled 1/3 cup low-sodium vegetable broth 2¾ cups fresh baby spinach
- 2 teaspoons low-sodium soy sauce
- 1 teaspoon ground turmeric
- 1 teaspoon fresh lemon juice

Instructions:

1.In a frying pan, heat the olive oil over medium-high heat and sauté the garlic for about 1 minute

2.Add the tofu and cook for about 3-4 minutes, slowly adding the broth.

3.Add the spinach, soy sauce and turmeric and stir fry for about 3-4 minutes or until all the liquid is absorbed

4.Remove and whisk in the lemon juice from the sun.

Tofu & Veggie Scramble

Prep Time: 15 minutes

Cook Time: 15 minutes

Serve: 2

Ingredients:

- ½ tablespoon olive oil
- 1 small onion, chopped finely
- 1 small red-bell-pepper, seeded and chopped finely
- 1 cup cherry tomatoes, chopped finely
- 1½ cups firm tofu, crumbled and chopped Pinch of cayenne pepper
- Pinch of ground turmeric
- Sea salt, to taste

Instructions:

1.In a skillet, heat-oil over medium-heat and sauté the onion and bell pepper for about 4-5 minutes.

2.Add the tomatoes and cook for about 1-2 minutes.

3.Add the tofu, turmeric, cayenne pepper and salt and cook for about 6-8 minutes.

Chicken & Zucchini Pancakes

Prep Time: 15 minutes

Cook Time: 32 minutes

Serve: 4

Ingredients:

- 4 cups zucchinis, shredded
- Salt, as required
- ¼ cup cooked chicken, shredded
- ¼ cup scallion, chopped finely
- 1 egg, beaten
- ¼ cup coconut flour
- Salt and ground-black-pepper, as required 1 tablespoon extra-virgin olive oil

Instructions:

1. In a colander, place the zucchini and sprinkle with salt.

2. Set aside for about 8-10 minutes.

3. Squeeze the zucchinis well and transfer into a bowl.

4. In the bowl of zucchini, add the remaining ingredients and mix until well combined.

5.Heat the oil in a big-nonstick skillet over normal heat.

6.Add ¼ cup of zucchini mixture into the preheated skillet and spread in an even layer.

7.Cook for about 3-4 minutes per side.

8.Repeat with the remaining mixture.

Broccoli Waffles

Prep Time: 10 minutes

Cook Time: 8 minutes

Serve: 2

Ingredients:

- 1/3 cup broccoli, chopped finely
- ¼ cup low-fat Cheddar cheese, shredded 1 egg
- ½ teaspoon garlic powder
- ½ teaspoon dried onion, minced
- Salt and ground black pepper, as required

Instructions:

1.Preheat a mini waffle iron and then grease it.

2.In a normal bowl, place all ingredients and mix until well combined.

3.Place ½ of the mixture into preheated waffle iron and cook for about 3-4 minutes or until golden brown.

4.Repeat with the remaining mixture.

Cheesy Spinach Waffles

Prep Time: 10 minutes

Cook Time: 20 minutes

Serve: 4

Ingredients:

- 1 large egg, beaten
- 1 cup ricotta cheese, crumbled
- ½ cup part-skim Mozzarella cheese, shredded
- ¼ cup low-fat Parmesan cheese, grated
- 4 ounces frozen-spinach, thawed and squeezed dry
- 1 garlic clove, minced
- Salt and ground black pepper, as required

Instructions:

1. Preheat a mini waffle iron and then grease it.

2. Stir in all the ingredients in a bowl and beat until well mixed.

3. Place ¼ of the mixture into preheated waffle iron and cook for about 4-5 minutes or until golden brown. Repeat with the remaining mixture.

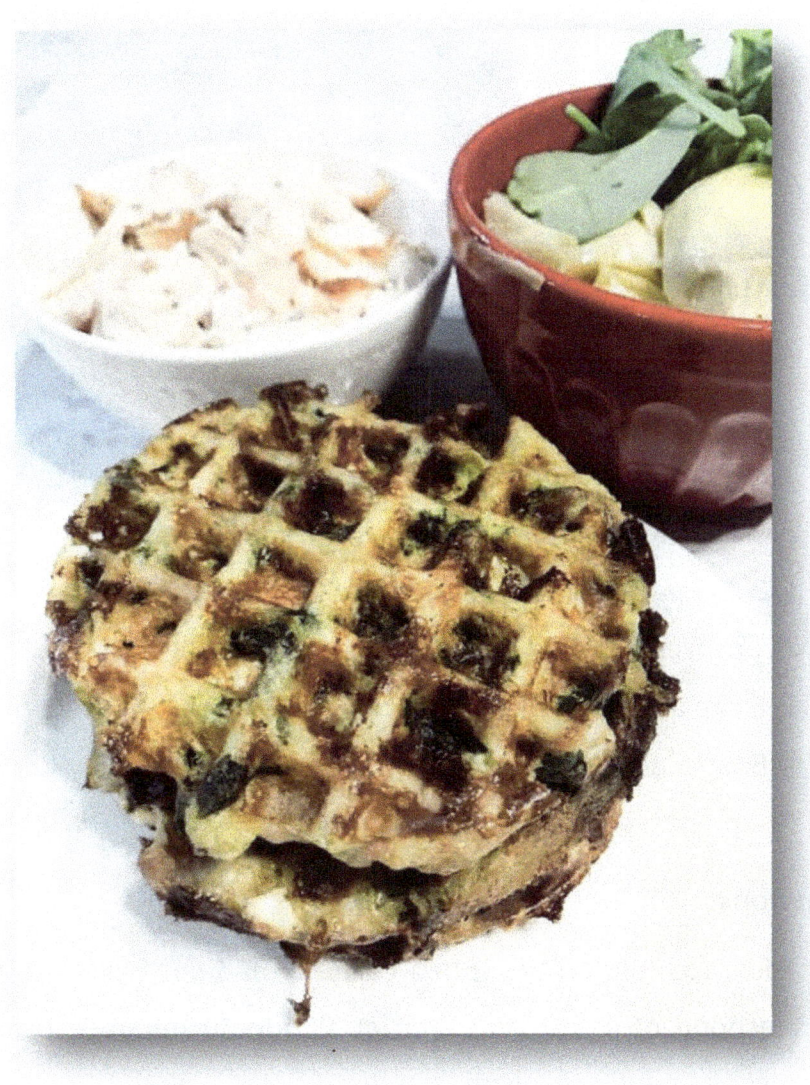

Pesto Zucchini Noodles

Time: 30 minutes

Serve: 4

Ingredients:

- 4 zucchini, spiralized
- 1 tbsp avocado oil
- 2 garlic cloves, chopped
- 2/3 cup olive oil
- 1/3 cup parmesan cheese, grated
- 2 cups fresh basil
- 1/3 cup almonds
- 1/8 tsp black pepper
- ¾ tsp sea salt

Instructions:

1. Add zucchini noodles into a colander and sprinkle with ¼ teaspoon of salt. Cover and let sit for 30 minutes. Drain zucchini noodles well and pat dry.
2. Preheat the oven to 400 F.

3. Place almonds on a parchment-lined baking sheet and bake for 6-8 minutes. Transfer toasted almonds into the food processor and process until coarse.

4. Add olive oil, cheese, basil, garlic, pepper, and remaining salt in a food processor with almonds and process until pesto texture.

5. Heat the avocado-oil in a pan over medium to high heat. Add zucchini noodles and cook for 4-5 minutes.

6. Pour pesto over zucchini noodles, mix well and cook for 1 minute.

7. Serve immediately with baked salmon.

Nutrition: Calories 525 Fat 47.4 g Carbs 9.3 g Sugar 3.8 g Protein 16.6 g Cholesterol 30 mg

Baked Cod & Vegetables

Time: 30 minutes

Serve: 4

Ingredients:

- 1 lb cod fillets
- 8 oz asparagus, chopped
- 3 cups broccoli, chopped
- ¼ cup parsley, minced
- ½ tsp lemon pepper seasoning
- ½ tsp paprika
- ¼ cup olive oil
- ¼ cup lemon juice
- 1 tsp salt

Instructions:

Preheat the oven to 410 F. Cover the pan with baking paper and

1. Set aside.

2. In a small bowl, mix lemon juice, paprika, olive oil, lemon pepper seasoning, and salt.

3. Place fish fillets in the middle of the parchment paper. Place broccoli and asparagus around the fish fillets.

4. Pour lemon juice mixture over the fish fillets and top with parsley.

5. Bake in preheated oven for 13-15 minutes.

Nutrition: Calories 240 Fat 14.1 g Carbs 7.6 g Sugar 2.6 g Protein 23.7 g Cholesterol 56 mg

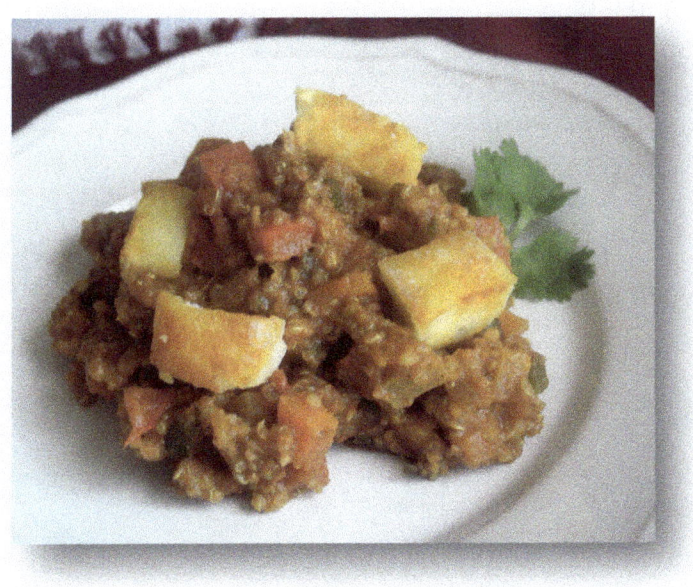

Parmesan Zucchini

Time: 30 minutes

Serve: 4

Ingredients:

- 4 zucchini, quartered lengthwise
- 2 tbsp fresh parsley, chopped
- 2 tbsp olive oil
- ¼ tsp garlic powder
- ½ tsp dried basil
- ½ tsp dried oregano
- ½ tsp dried thyme
- ½ cup parmesan cheese, grated
- Pepper
- Salt

Instructions:

1.Preheat the oven to 355 F. Line baking sheet with parchment paper and set aside.

2.In a small bowl, mix parmesan cheese, garlic powder, basil, oregano, thyme, pepper, and salt.

3.Arrange zucchini onto the prepared baking sheet and drizzle with oil and sprinkle with parmesan cheese mixture.

4. Cook for 16 minutes in a preheated oven, then broil for 2 minutes or until lightly browned.

5.Garnish with parsley and serve immediately.

Nutrition: Calories 244 Fat 16.4 g Carbs 7 g Sugar 3.5 g Protein 14.5 g Cholesterol 30 mg

Chicken Zucchini Noodles

Time: 25 minutes

Serve: 2

Ingredients:

- 1 large zucchini, spiralized
- 1 chicken breast, skinless & boneless
- ½ tbsp jalapeno, minced
- 2 garlic cloves, minced
- ½ tsp ginger, minced
- ½ tbsp fish sauce
- 2 tbsp coconut cream
- ½ tbsp honey
- ½ lime juice
- 1 tbsp peanut butter
- 1 carrot, chopped
- 2 tbsp cashews, chopped
- ¼ cup fresh cilantro, chopped
- 1 tbsp olive oil
- Pepper
- Salt

Instructions:

Heat the olive oil in a pan.

1. Season chicken breast with pepper and salt. Add the chicken breast to the pan once the oil is hot and cook for 3-4 minutes on each side or until cooked.

2. Remove chicken breast from pan. Shred chicken breast with a fork and set aside.

3. In a small bowl, mix peanut butter, jalapeno, garlic, ginger, fish sauce, coconut cream, honey, and lime juice. Set aside.

4. In a large mixing bowl, combine spiralized zucchini, carrots, cashews, cilantro, and shredded chicken.

5. Pour peanut butter mixture over zucchini noodles and toss to combine.

Nutrition: Calories 353 Fat 21.1 g Carbs 20.5 g Sugar 10.8 g Protein 24.5 g Cholesterol 54 mg

Tomato Cucumber Avocado Salad

Time: 15 minutes

Serve: 4

Ingredients:

- 12 oz cherry tomatoes, cut in half
- 5 small cucumbers, chopped
- 3 small avocados, chopped
- ½ tsp ground black pepper
- 2 tbsp olive oil
- 2 tbsp fresh lemon juice
- ¼ cup fresh cilantro, chopped
- 1 tsp sea salt

Instructions:

1. Add cherry tomatoes, cucumbers, avocados, and cilantro into the large mixing bowl and mix well.

2. Mix olive oil, lemon juice, black pepper, and salt and pour over salad.

3. Toss well and serve immediately.

Nutrition: Calories 442 Fat 37.1 g Carbs 30.3 g Sugar 9.4 g Protein 6.2 g Cholesterol 0 mg

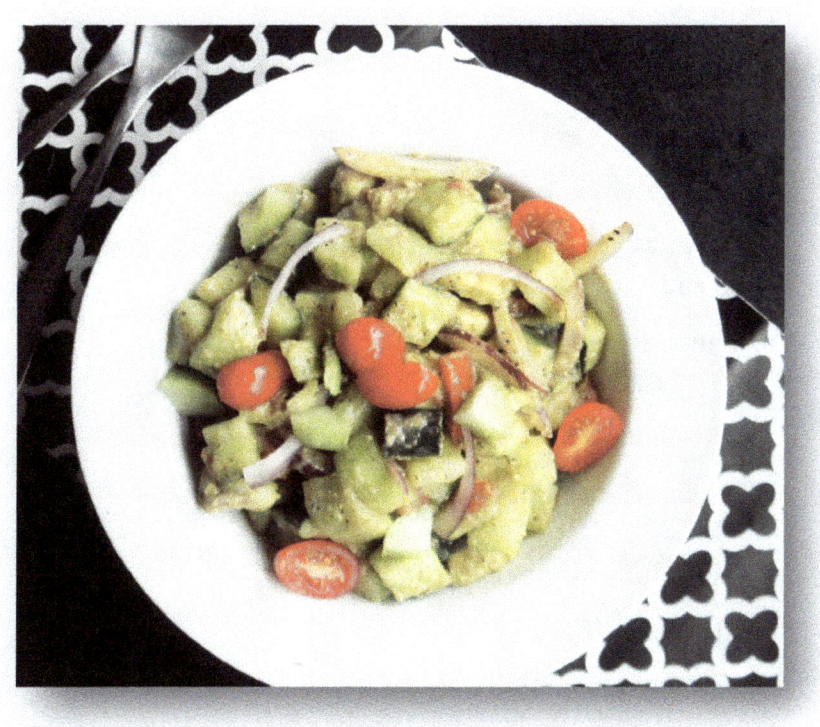

Creamy Cauliflower Soup

Time: 30 minutes

Serve: 6

Ingredients:

- 5 cups cauliflower rice
- 8 oz cheddar cheese, grated
- 2 cups unsweetened almond milk
- 2 cups vegetable stock
- 2 tbsp water
- 1 small onion, chopped
- 2 garlic cloves, minced
- 1 tbsp olive oil
- Pepper
- Salt

Instructions:

1. Heat olive-oil over medium heat in a big stockpot.

2. Add onion and garlic and cook for 1-2 minutes.

3. Add cauliflower rice and water. Cover and cook for 5-7 minutes.

3. Now add vegetable stock and almond milk and stir well. Bring to boil.

4.Turn heat to low and simmer for 5 minutes.

5.Turn off the heat. Slowly add cheddar cheese and stir until smooth.

6.Season soup with pepper and salt.

7.Stir well and serve hot.

Nutrition: Calories 214 Fat 16.5 g Carbs 7.3 g Sugar 3 g Protein 11.6 g Cholesterol 40 mg

Taco Zucchini Boats

Time: 70 minutes

Serve: 4

Ingredients:

- 4 medium zucchinis, cut in half lengthwise
- ¼ cup fresh cilantro, chopped
- ½ cup cheddar cheese, shredded
- ¼ cup of water
- 4 oz tomato sauce
- 2 tbsp bell pepper, mined
- ½ small onion, minced
- ½ tsp oregano
- 1 tsp paprika
- 1 tsp chili powder
- 1 tsp cumin
- 1 tsp garlic powder
- 1 lb lean ground turkey
- ½ cup of salsa
- 1 tsp kosher salt

Instructions:

1. Preheat the oven to 400 F.

2. Add ¼ cup of salsa to the bottom of the baking dish.

3. Using a spoon, hollow out the center of the zucchini halves.

4. Chop the scooped-out flesh of zucchini and set aside ¾ of a cup of chopped flesh.

5. Add zucchini halves to the boiling water and cook for 1 minute. Remove zucchini halves from water.

6. Add ground turkey in a large pan and cook until meat is no longer pink. Add spices and mix well.

7. Add reserved zucchini flesh, water, tomato sauce, bell pepper, and onion. Stir well and cover, simmer over low heat for 20 minutes.

8. Stuff zucchini boats with taco meat and top each with one tablespoon of shredded cheddar cheese.

9. Place zucchini boats in a baking dish. Cover the dish with paper and bake in a preheated oven

    1. 35 minutes.

    2. Top with remaining salsa and chopped cilantro.

Nutrition: Calories 297 Fat 13.7 g Carbs 17.2 g Sugar 9.3 g Protein 30.2 g Cholesterol 96 mg

Healthy Broccoli Salad

Time: 25 minutes

Serve: 6

Ingredients:

- 3 cups broccoli, chopped
- 1 tbsp apple cider vinegar
- ½ cup Greek yogurt
- 2 tbsp sunflower seeds
- 3 bacon slices, cooked and chopped
- 1/3 cup onion, sliced
- ¼ tsp stevia

Instructions:

1. In a mixing bowl, mix broccoli, onion, and bacon.

2. In a small bowl, mix yogurt, vinegar, and stevia and pour over broccoli mixture. Stir to combine.

3. Sprinkle sunflower seeds on top of the salad.

4. Store salad in the refrigerator for 30 minutes.

Nutrition: Calories 90 Fat 4.9 g Carbs 5.4 g Sugar 2.5 g Protein 6.2 g Cholesterol 12 mg

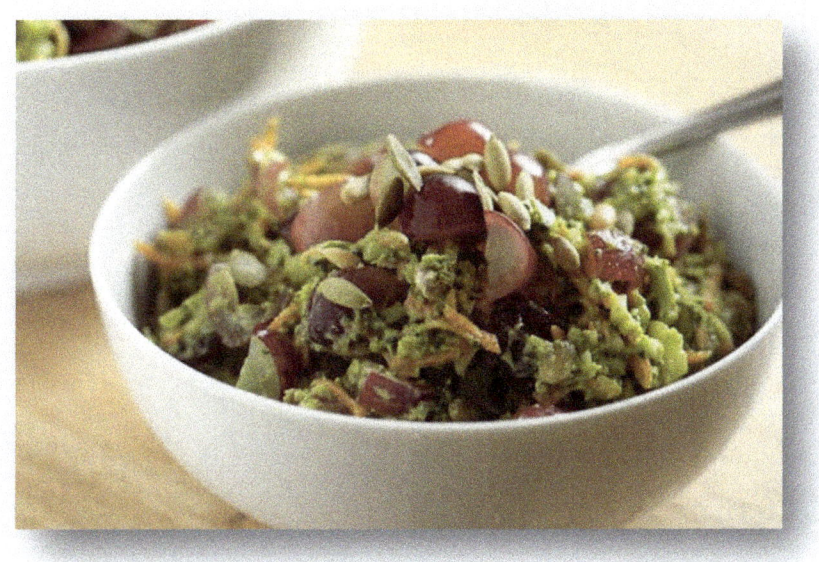

Delicious Zucchini Quiche

Time: 60 minutes

Serve: 8

Ingredients:

- 6 eggs
- 2 medium zucchini, shredded
- ½ tsp dried basil
- 2 garlic cloves, minced
- 1 tbsp dry onion, minced
- 2 tbsp parmesan cheese, grated
- 2 tbsp fresh parsley, chopped
- ½ cup olive oil
- 1 cup cheddar cheese, shredded
- ¼ cup coconut flour
- ¾ cup almond flour
- ½ tsp salt

Instructions:

1. Preheat the furnace to 355 F. Grease a 9-inch dish of pie and set aside.

2. Squeeze out excess liquid from zucchini.

3. Into the cup, add all ingredients and blend until well mixed. Pour into the prepared pie dish.

4. Bake in preheated oven for 47-63 minutes or until set.

5. Remove it from the oven and let it cool down completely.

Nutrition: Calories 288 Fat 26.3 g Carbs 5 g Sugar 1.6 g Protein 11 g Cholesterol 139 mg

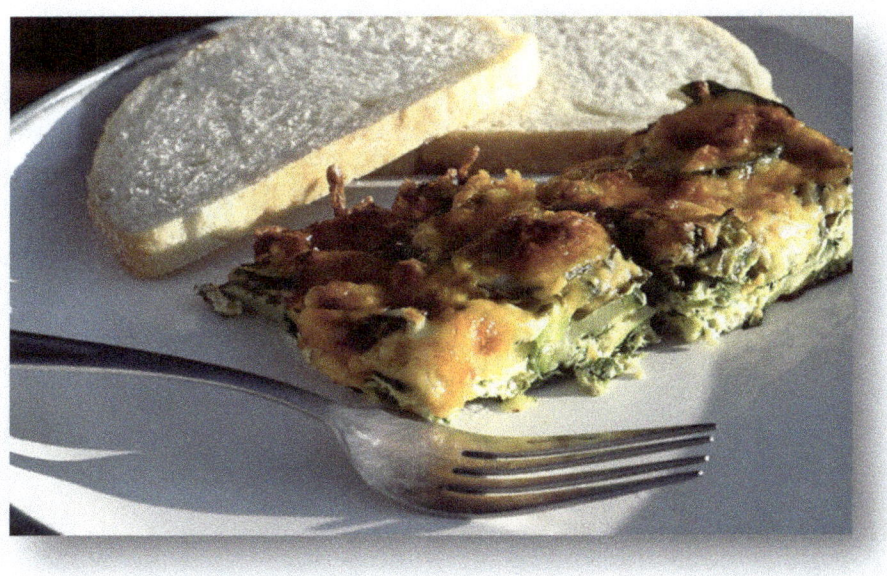

Turkey Spinach Egg Muffins

Time: 30 minutes

Serve: 3

Ingredients:

- 5 egg whites
- 2 eggs
- ¼ cup cheddar cheese, shredded
- ¼ cup spinach, chopped
- ¼ cup milk
- 3 lean breakfast turkey sausage
- Pepper
- Salt

Instructions:

1. Preheat the oven to 355 F. Grease muffin tray cups and set aside.

2. In a pan, brown the turkey sausage links over medium-high heat until the sausage is brown from all the sides.

3. Cut sausage into ½-inch pieces and set aside.

4.In a big bowl, whisk together eggs, egg whites, milk, pepper, and salt. Stir in spinach.

5.Pour egg mixture into the prepared muffin tray.

6.Divide sausage and cheese evenly between each muffin cup.

7.Bake in a preheated oven for 22 minutes or until muffins are set.

Nutrition: Calories 123 Fat 6.8 g Carbs 1.9 g Sugar 1.6 g Protein 13.3 g Cholesterol 123 mg

Chicken Casserole

Time: 40 minutes

Serve: 4

Ingredients:

- 1 lb cooked chicken, shredded
- ¼ cup Greek yogurt
- 1 cup cheddar cheese, shredded
- ½ cup of salsa
- 4 oz cream cheese, softened
- 4 cups cauliflower florets
- 1/8 tsp black pepper
- ½ tsp kosher salt

Instructions:

1. Add cauliflower florets into the microwave-safe dish and cook for 10 minutes or until tender.

2. Add cream cheese and microwave for 35 seconds more. Stir well.

3. Add chicken, yogurt, cheddar cheese, salsa, pepper, and salt, and stir everything well.

4. Preheat the oven to 375 F.

5.Bake in preheated oven for 20 minutes.

Nutrition: Calories 429 Fat 23 g Carbs 9.6 g Sugar 4.7 g Protein 45.4 g Cholesterol 149 mg

Shrimp Cucumber Salad

Time: 20 minutes

Serve: 4

Ingredients:

- 1 lb shrimp, cooked
- 1 bell pepper, sliced
- 2 green onions, sliced
- ½ cup fresh cilantro, chopped
- 2 cucumbers, sliced

For dressing:

- 2 tbsp fresh mint leaves, chopped
- 1 tsp sesame seeds
- ½ tsp red pepper flakes
- 1 tbsp olive oil
- ¼ cup rice wine vinegar
- ¼ cup lime juice
- 1 Serrano chili pepper, minced
- 3 garlic cloves, minced
- ½ tsp salt

Instructions:

1.In a little bowl, whisk together all dressing ingredients and set aside.

2.In a mixing bowl, mix shrimp, bell pepper, green onion, cilantro, and cucumbers.

3.Pour dressing over salad and toss well.

Nutrition: Calories 219 Fat 6.1 g Carbs 11.3 g Sugar 4.2 g Protein 27.7 g Cholesterol 239 mg

Asparagus & Shrimp Stir Fry

Time: 20 minutes

Serve: 4

Ingredients:

- 1 lb asparagus
- 1 lb shrimp
- 2 tbsp lemon juice
- 1 tbsp soy sauce
- 1 tsp ginger, minced
- 1 garlic clove, minced
- 1 tsp red pepper flakes
- ¼ cup olive oil
- Pepper and Salt

Instructions:

1. Heat 2 normal spoons of oil in a large pan over medium-high heat.

2. Add shrimp to the pan and season with red pepper flakes, pepper, salt, and cook for 5 minutes.

3. Remove shrimp from pan and set aside.

4.Add remaining oil in the same pan. Add garlic, ginger, and asparagus, stir frequently, and cook until asparagus is tender about 5 minutes.

5.Return shrimp to the pan. Add lemon-juice and soy-sauce and stir until well combined.

Nutrition: Calories 274 Fat 14.8 g Carbs 7.4 g Sugar 2.4 g Protein 28.8 g Cholesterol 239 mg

Turkey Burgers

Time: 30 minutes

Serve: 4

Ingredients:

- 1 lb lean ground turkey
- 2 green onions, sliced
- ¼ cup basil leaves, shredded
- 2 garlic cloves, minced
- 2 medium zucchini, shredded and squeeze out all the liquid
- ½ tsp black pepper
- ½ tsp sea salt

Instructions:

1.Heat grill to medium heat.

2.To the cup, add all the ingredients and combine until well blended.

3.Make four equal shapes of patties from the mixture.

4.Spray one piece of foil with cooking spray.

5. Place prepared patties on the foil and grill for 10 minutes. Turn patties to the other side and grill for 10 minutes more.

Nutrition: Calories 183 Fat 8.3 g Carbs 4.5 g Sugar 1.9 g Protein 23.8 g Cholesterol 81 mg

Broccoli Kale Salmon Burgers

Time: 30 minutes

Serve: 5

Ingredients:

- 2 eggs
- ½ cup onion, chopped
- ½ cup broccoli, chopped
- ½ cup kale, chopped
- ½ tsp garlic powder
- 2 tbsp lemon juice
- ½ cup almond flour
- 15 oz can salmon, drained and bones removed
- ½ tsp salt

Instructions:

1.Line one plate with parchment paper and set aside.

2.Add all ingredients into the big bowl and mix until well combined.

3.Make five equal shapes of patties from the mixture and place them on a prepared plate.

4.Place plate in the refrigerator for 30 minutes.

5.Spray a big pan with cooking spray and heat over medium heat.

6.Once the pan is hot, then add patties and cook for 5-7 minutes per side.

Nutrition: Calories 221 Fat 12.6 g Carbs 5.2 g Sugar 1.4 g Protein 22.1 g Cholesterol 112 mg

Pan Seared Cod

Time: 25 minutes

Serve: 4

Ingredients:

- 1 ¾ lbs cod fillets
- 1 tbsp ranch seasoning
- 4 tsp olive oil

Instructions:

1.Heat oil in a big pan over medium-high heat.

2.Season fish fillets with ranch seasoning.

3.Once the oil is hot, then place fish fillets in a pan and cook for 6-8 minutes on each side.

Nutrition: Calories 207 Fat 6.4 g Carbs 0 g Sugar 0 g Protein 35.4 g Cholesterol 97 mg

Quick Lemon Pepper Salmon

Time: 18 minutes

Serve: 4

Ingredients:

- 1 ½ lbs salmon fillets
- ½ tsp ground black pepper
- 1 tsp dried oregano
- 2 garlic cloves, minced
- ¼ cup olive oil
- 1 lemon juice
- 1 tsp sea salt

Instructions:

1. In a big bowl, mix lemon-juice, olive-oil, garlic, oregano, black pepper, and salt.

2. Add fish fillets in the bowl and coat well with the marinade, and place in the refrigerator for 15 minutes.

3. Preheat the grill.

4. Brush grill grates with oil.

5.Place marinated salmon fillets on hot grill and cook for 4 minutes, then turn salmon fillets to the other side and cook for 4 minutes more.

Nutrition: Calories 340 Fat 23.3 g Carbs 1.2 g Sugar 0.3 g Protein 33.3 g Cholesterol 75 mg

Healthy Salmon Salad

Time: 20 minutes

Serve: 2

Ingredients:

- 2 salmon fillets
- 2 tbsp olive oil
- ¼ cup onion, chopped
- 1 cucumber, peeled and sliced
- 1 avocado, diced
- 2 tomatoes, chopped
- 4 cups baby spinach
- Pepper and Salt

Instructions:

1.Heat the olive oil in a pan.

2.Season salmon fillets with pepper and salt. Place fish fillets in a pan and cook for 4-5 minutes.

3.Turn fish fillets and cook for 2-3 minutes more.

4.Divide remaining ingredients evenly between two bowls, then top with cooked fish fillet.

Nutrition: Calories 350 Fat 23.2 g Carbs 15.3 g Sugar 6.6 g Protein 25 g Cholesterol 18 mg

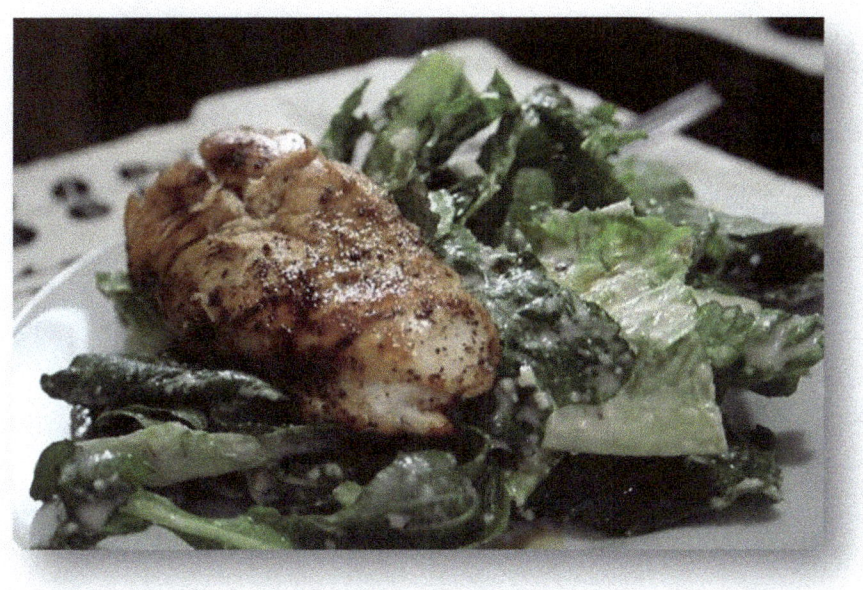

Pan Seared Tilapia

Time: 18 minutes

Serve: 2

Ingredients:

- 18 oz tilapia fillets
- ¼ tsp lemon pepper
- ½ tsp parsley flakes
- ¼ tsp garlic powder
- 1 tsp Cajun seasoning
- ½ tsp dried oregano
- 2 tbsp olive oil

Instructions:

1. Heat the olive oil in a pan.

2. Season fish fillets with lemon pepper, parsley flakes, garlic powder, Cajun seasoning, and oregano.

3. Place fish fillets in the pan and cook for 3-4 minutes on each side.

Nutrition: Calories 333 Fat 16.4 g Carbs 0.7 g Sugar 0.1 g Protein 47.6 g Cholesterol 124 mg

Creamy Broccoli Soup

Time: 35 minutes

Serve: 8

Ingredients:

- 20 oz frozen broccoli, thawed and chopped
- ¼ tsp nutmeg
- 4 cups vegetable broth
- 1 potato, peeled and chopped
- 2 garlic cloves, peeled and chopped
- 1 large onion, chopped
- 1 tbsp olive oil
- Pepper and Salt

Instructions:

1. Heat the olive oil in a pan.

2. Add the onion, garlic and sauté until the onion is tender.

3. Add potato, broccoli, and broth and bring to boil. Turn heat to low and simmer for 15 minutes or until vegetables are tender.

4.Using a blender, puree the soup until smooth. Season soup with nutmeg, pepper, and salt.

Nutrition: Calories 84 Fat 2.7 g Carbs 10.9 g Sugar 2.6 g Protein 5.1 g Cholesterol 0 mg

Tuna Muffins

Time: 35 minutes

Serve: 8

Ingredients:

- 2 eggs, lightly beaten
- 1 can tuna, flaked
- 1 tsp cayenne pepper
- 1/4 cup mayonnaise
- 1 celery stalk, chopped
- 1 1/2 cups cheddar cheese, shredded
- 1/4 cup sour cream
- Pepper and Salt

Instructions:

1.Preheat the oven to 355 F. Grease muffin tin and set aside.

2.Add all ingredients into the big bowl and mix until well combined, and pour into the prepared muffin tin.

3.Bake for 25 minutes.

Nutrition: Calories 185 Fat 14 g Carbs 2.6 g Sugar 0.7 g Protein 13 g Cholesterol 75 mg

Chicken Cauliflower Rice

Time: 25 minutes

Serve: 4

Ingredients:

- 1 cauliflower head, chopped
- 2 cups cooked chicken, shredded
- 1 tsp olive oil
- 1 tsp garlic powder
- 1 tsp chili powder
- 1 tsp cumin
- 1/4 cup tomatoes, diced
- Salt

Instructions:

1.Add cauliflower into the food processor and process until you get rice size pieces.

2.Heat oil in a pan over high heat.

3.Add cauliflower rice and chicken in a pan and cook for 5-7 minutes.

4.Add garlic powder, chili powder, cumin, tomatoes, and salt. Stir well and cook for 7-10 minutes more.

Nutrition: Calories 140 Fat 3.6 g Carbs 5 g Sugar 2 g Protein 22 g Cholesterol 54 mg

Easy Spinach Muffins

Time: 25 minutes

Serve: 12

Ingredients:

- 10 eggs
- 2 cups spinach, chopped
- 1/4 tsp garlic powder
- 1/4 tsp onion powder
- 1/2 tsp dried basil
- 1 1/2 cups parmesan cheese, grated
- Salt

Instructions:

1.Preheat the oven to 410 F. Grease muffin tin and set aside.

2.In a large bowl, whisk eggs with basil, garlic powder, onion powder, and salt.

3.Add cheese and spinach and stir well.

4.Pour egg-mixture into the prepared muffin tin and bake 15 minutes.

Nutrition: Calories 110 Fat 7 g Carbs 1 g Sugar 0.3 g Protein 9 g Cholesterol 165 mg

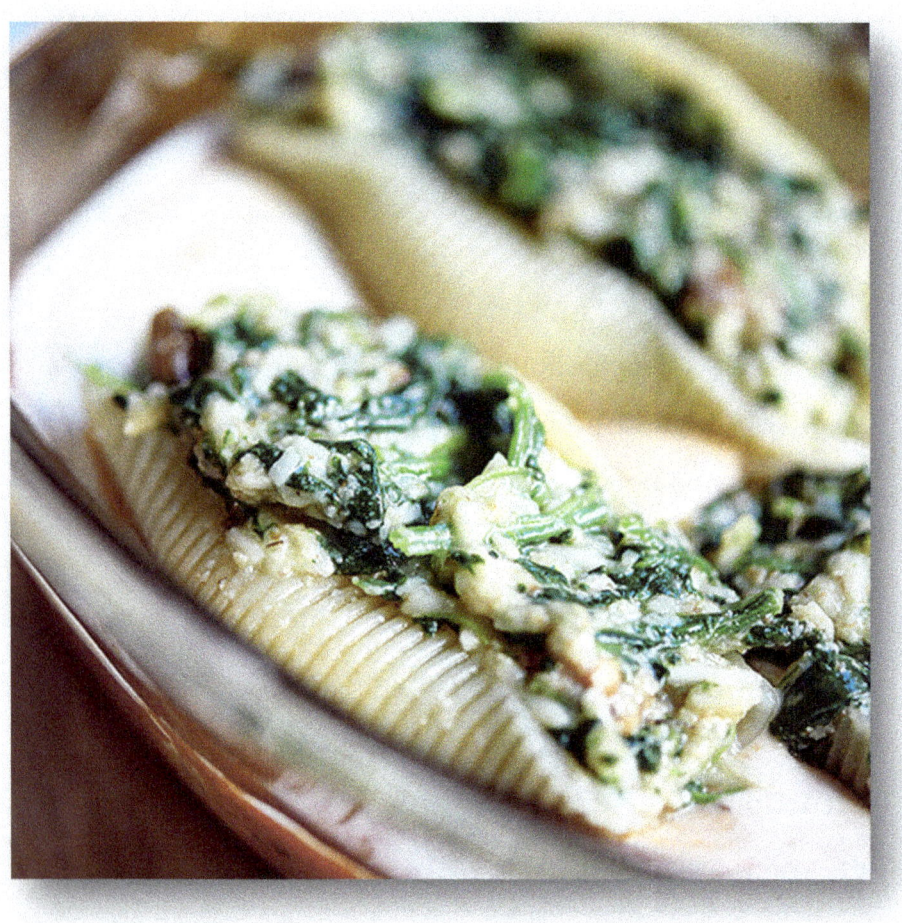

Healthy Cauliflower Grits

Time: 2 hours 10 minutes

Serve: 8

Ingredients:

- 6 cups cauliflower rice
- 1/4 tsp garlic powder
- 1 cup cream cheese
- 1/2 cup vegetable stock
- 1/4 tsp onion powder
- 1/2 tsp pepper
- 1 tsp salt

Instructions:

1. Add all the ingredients to the slow-cooker and blend well.

2. Cover and cook on low for 2 hours.

Nutrition: Calories 126 Fat 10 g Carbs 5 g Sugar 2 g Protein 4 g Cholesterol 31 mg

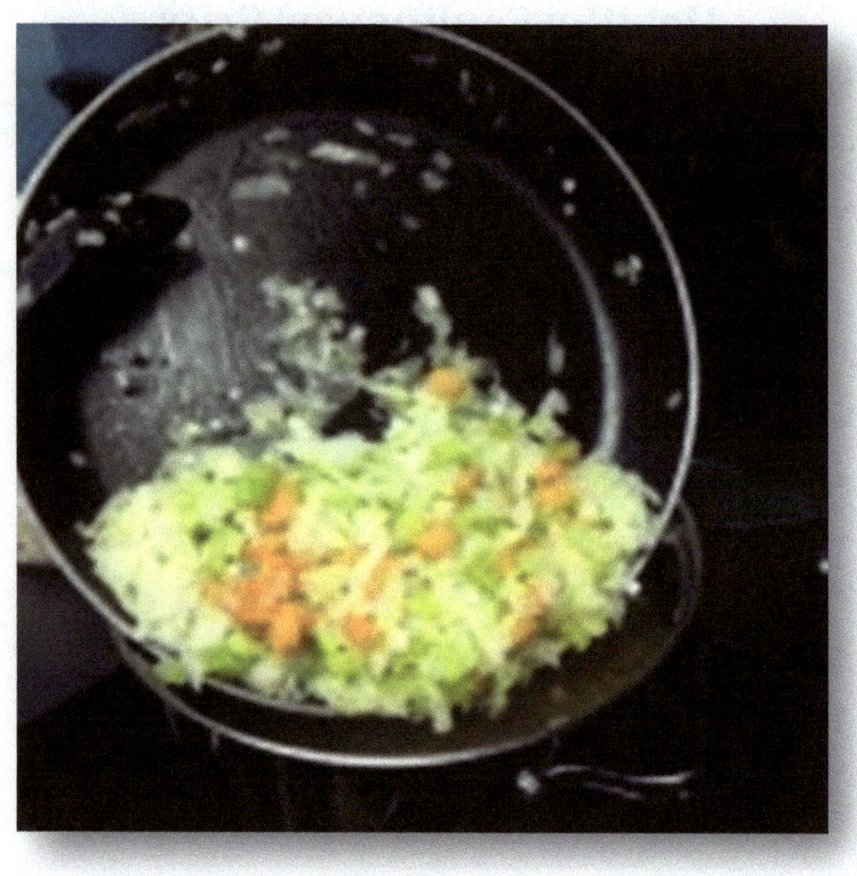

Spinach Tomato Frittata

Time: 30 minutes

Serve: 8

Ingredients:

- 12 eggs
- 2 cups baby spinach, shredded
- 1/4 cup sun-dried tomatoes, sliced
- 1/2 tsp dried basil
- 1/4 cup parmesan cheese, grated
- Pepper and Salt

Instructions:

1. Preheat the oven to 425 F. Grease oven-safe pan and set aside.

2. In a large bowl, whisk eggs with pepper and salt. Add remaining ingredients and stir to combine.

3. Pour egg-mixture into the prepared pan and bake for 20 minutes.

Nutrition: Calories 116 Fat 7 g Carbs 1 g Sugar 1 g Protein 10 g Cholesterol 250 mg

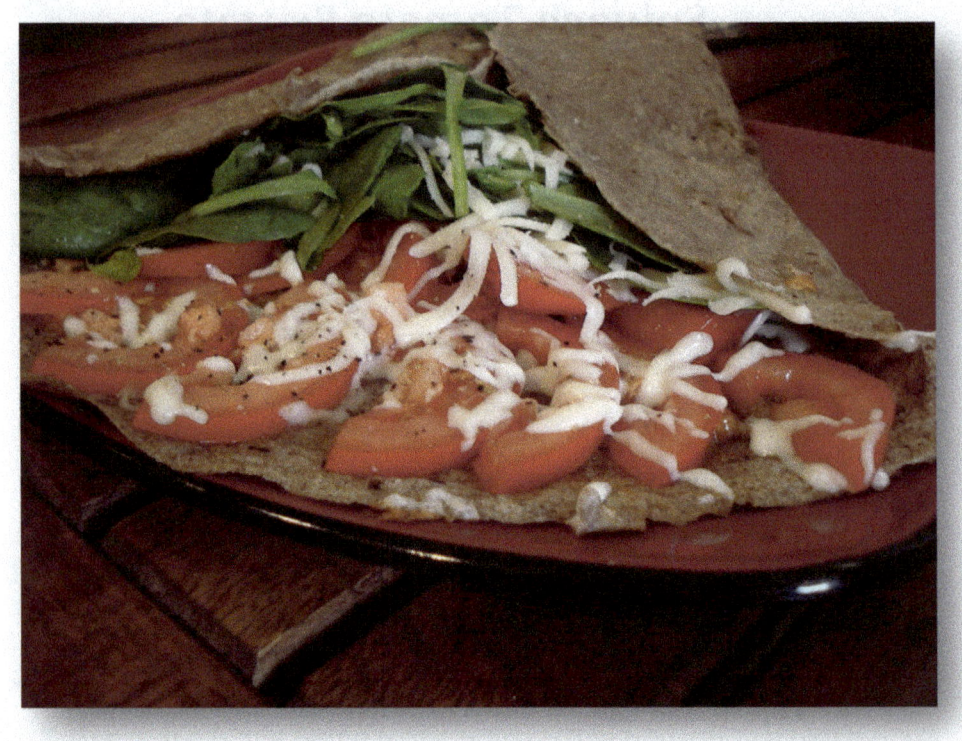